More Massages Please!

Massage with a Legal Hand Release

By Phila Vocia

Before you shake your head or run away,

consider these few points:

Biology, the study of how natural elements combine

Anatomy, the study of your physical form

Sociology, the study of people interacting

Anthropology, the study of learned behavior

Survival, the uncanny ability that through selection a person, thing or idea stays worthy and with life in it.

The time has come we need a legal hand release situation.

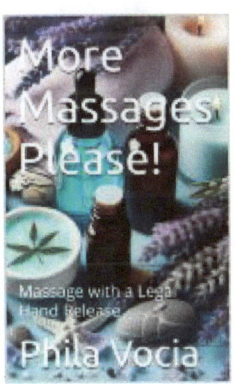

Printer Info

Front and Back cover Illustrations were designed by Phila Vocia.

This is an Amazon Kindle Book.

Available at the Kindle Books section at Amazon
www.amazon.com

FEEL FREE TO SHARE ANY PHOTO OR PORTION OF THIS BOOK. HOWEVER, FOR GIVING AS A GIFT IT'S BEST TO PURCHASE THE WHOLE BOOK AND SEND IT. Front and back cover Illustrations are designed by Phila Vocia

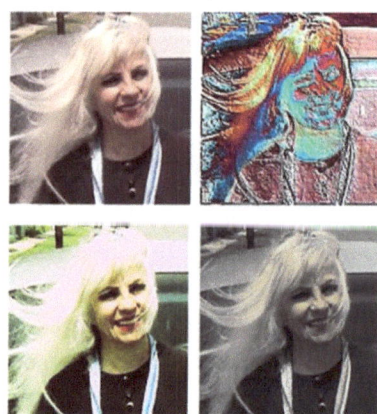

Disclaimer

The information depicted on the pages within this book is strictly representing hypothetical situations.

None of the recommendations are made to offend or are they a promise. It is up to the reader to make their own opinion and perhaps get involved at the Local, State or National level to make a change.

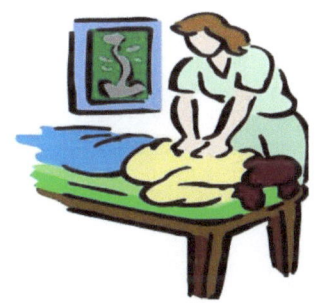

Dedication

After more than 20 years in the sex industry, trying just about all of it except for the most eccentric, my conclusions are based on real life experiences while listening to the concerns of clients, noting the heart ache from the religious in marriages that are stifled and devoid from sex, the worry of women who wonder will my mate come home, the relief of the not so perfect, disabled, hard to date and otherwise awfully lonely who reach out for comfort, the satisfaction of the healthy, wealthy and wise when they get what they need then walk away as easy as getting off a bus.

This is for all of you so we, the experienced, can pass on the knowledge.

Contents

The theme is to encourage society to legalize a hand release. To stop people from massaging in cars, boats, trucks and public bathrooms, public outdoor areas, etc. we should set the law books straight from the beginning. If we set the verbiage in the laws books to read: **A hand release is legal when it is included in a massage situation in a massage parlor, salon, spa or fitness center. And we need a separate category for Body Rub people with perhaps less training required and who would also be able to give a hand release.**

Images: Color Images, Other Images,

The End Page: Website Information

Preface

As mankind evolved, they cared about their immediate family, you know, their loins, their own blood. Then a business and wealth evolved they cared about the inheritance they would leave to their children. We can't be so consumed with what we are leaving our children as to blow up the planet over it.

We feel that the contents of this book are useful in any country. Tell your friends that we can make the massage industry more exciting, while keeping families safe too.

Stay safe and enjoy.

Phila Vocia, Author

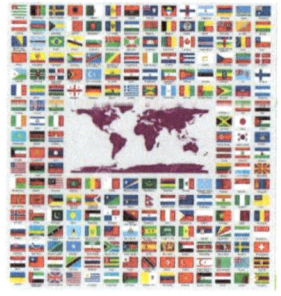

Overview

The best place to get the dialogue started is with the current college students. Day by day we will contact their groups and clubs and encourage them to start debates and podcasts. If you see, any be sure to make a comment, like or even send them a donation.

Seek others who are talking about this idea. Cast an Anonymous Vote, Disscusion is important..

If a body rub can be a separate category and include an option legal hand release, it would solve many problems for men and women.

Make getting a hand release a common activity and leave the muscle and joint healing to the masseuses, who are often times, paid by insurance companies.

Sometimes a client wants a choice.

"Booya," also spelled "Booyah," is used as an interjection to signal satisfaction or accomplishment. We all need more Booya!

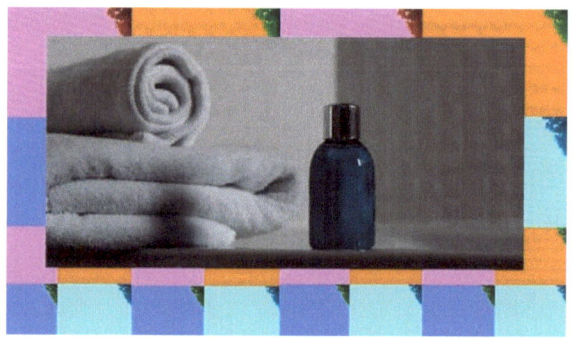

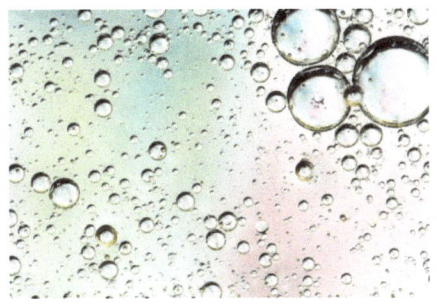

My name is Phila Vocia.

I wrote 2 books on Amazon Kindle to promote the possibility of legalizing a hand release, or a self pleasure ending, for men and women who are over 18 years of age.

I created a website and took a poll. It talked about legalizing a hand release inside of a massage situation. (We listed the Rigor and Renew domain for sale on April 06, 2025)

Our Visitor Count

001084

They Voted Anonymously!

Nonprofit wishes to help Legalize a Hand Release in a Salon or Studio

Results

3 Questions

Yes or No Answers

Make Body Rub Workers a different job category from Licensed Masseuses?

Make it legal that a Massage or Body Rub can optionally include a hand release?

Would you still get regular or therapeutic massages if body rubs with hand releases are offered?

There were more Yes votes to all three questions

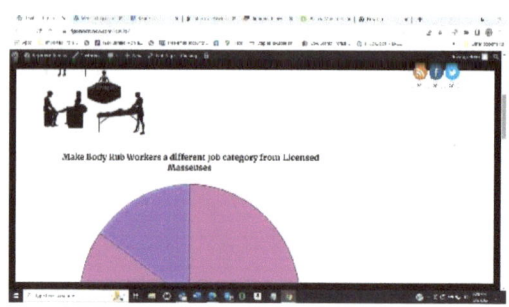

You are encouraged to make your own poll and get answers on this up-and-coming topic.

Sponsored by: Wellspring Relief a NJ Nonprofit Corporation, Mailing Address: P O Box 5233, Atlantic City, NJ 08401 https://www.wellspringrelief.org/

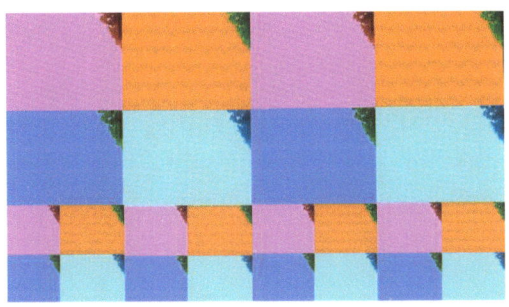

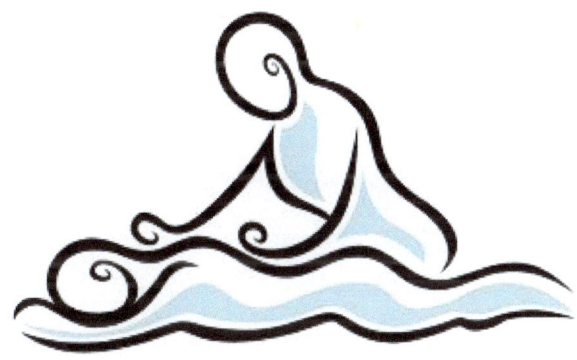

Make it Safer

Like shark fishing, sky diving and anything else that can be dangerous, Independent Body Rubs and Massage Outcalls can be dangerous if you meet up with a person who has a criminal motive.

The clients worry too if the worker is going to be courteous, kind and polite, do a good job and leave peacefully and not set up to do any criminal activity after the appointment.

Real life experiences while listening to the concerns of clients, many people know of the heart ache from the religious men in marriages that are stifled and devoid from sex, the worry couples face who wonder will my mate come home if he has an encounter. And realizing the relief of the not so perfect, disabled, hard to date and otherwise awfully lonely, who reach out for comfort. Then there is the entire mainstream to consider, the satisfaction of the healthy, wealthy and wise, when they get what they need, then walk away as easy as getting off a bus.

The best place to get the dialogue started is with the current college students. Day by day we will contact their groups and clubs and encourage them to start debates and podcasts. If you see, any be sure to make a comment, like or even send them a donation.

WITH THE ABOVE BEING SAID, MAKE A HAND RELEASE LEGAL FOR BODY RUB WORKERS AND MASSEUSES TO PROVIDE A HAND RELEASE TO CLIENTS THAT ARE OVER 18, QUALIFIED AS BEING PROVIDED INSIDE OF A SALON, STUDIO OR MASSAGE PARLOR. MILLIONS OF PEOPLE WILL BLOG, WRITE ARTICLES AND MAKE IT A SAFER INDUSTRY.

MILLIONS OF JOBS WILL BE CREATED AND MILLIONS OF TAX REVENUE WILL BE ACCOUNTED FOR. MILLIONS OF HAPPY PEOPLE WILL ENJOY THE SERVICES. PLEASE ASK YOUR CONGRESS MAN OR WOMAN TO HELP.

THESE STATES HAVE TRIED AND MAY TRY AGAIN. WASHINGTON DC, NEW YORK, CALIFORNIA, VERMONT AND MAINE. MORE STATES SHOULD MOVE FORWARD WITH THE BILLS AND PASS THEM.

CANADA HAS LEGALIZED SEX WORK IN SOME PROVINCES.

WE JUST WANT TO LEGALIZE THE HAND RELEASE.

THE TIMES THEY ARE A CHANGING. SHARE THIS WEBSITE AND THE BLOG ABOVE SO WE CAN BUILD OUR STATISTICS TO PRESENT TO LAWMAKERS.

MEN'S BIOLOGY IS IMPORTANT TO UNDERSTAND, AS MUCH AS IT IS TO UNDERSTAND A LADY'S.

HELP FIGHT PROCREATION PRESSURE!

LET'S VOTE FOR CHANGE SO ALL OF US CAN BE HAPPIER.

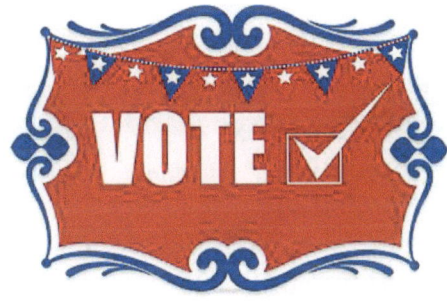

Here are 2 of my supportive websites.

Amazon Kindle
Phila Vocia Author Page Link
https://www.amazon.com/stores/author/B00MX1DI4Y/
Approx $2.99 More Massages Please! Massage with a Legal Hand Release
Approx $2.99 Massage with a Self Pleasure Ending

Rumble Modern Sexuality

https://rumble.com/c/c-1584695

Contact

Do you have a question, comment or do you want to help the cause?

Send an email to: info@wellspringrelief.org

Feeling Generous?

**Note: Hey friends! Surprise. Read all about it! Legalize a Hand Release inside of a massage situation. Make positive change for many, especially college students looking to start debates. Donate and share our cause with your network.
See our PayPal link at www.wellspringrelief.org**

Please contact me. I would like to speak with you about this cause. It is a timely concern for many people.
Phila Vocia
Wellspring Relief a NJ Nonprofit Corporation
info@wellspringrelief.org

Posted on September 8, 2020
Updated 04/06/2025

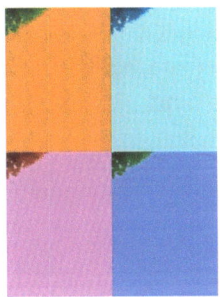

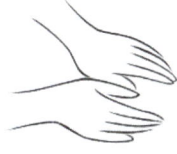

I am an American who believes in the separation of church and state. The religious leaders can argue all day about sex outside of marriage and some of their points are well taken since, the act of doing it often leads to false sexual highs and signals inducing a mate to leave their spouse for the new partner. These signals are false and temporary and often lead to the divorce or break up or separation or even just separate beds in the same home.

In this day and age of continuous stimulation from advertising not to mention the vast porn industry, all kinds of birth control available and the new generations having been exposed to this other era of products and services are expecting society to give them a legal answer to their biological needs that may not be met in a marriage or relationship.

Research shows that **men and women do go home to their mates, especially when the masseuse makes it clear that they are not interested in a relationship.**

A hand release is light action, non-emotional, it relieves the buildup in the man or woman and then they can get back to the activities of their daily life and visit with **and enjoy the people who are important to them.**

Everyone would be happy.

Yes, some people would push the folder and try to get phone numbers and meet elsewhere and do intense sex. If they are lucky, they can find out but mutually revealing that they are both not law enforcement. But you can be sure that the law enforcement people would be actively trying to find out if a man or woman is providing other services and they leave themselves open to arrests.

Arrests are terrible events in a person's life. It can lead to the loss of the mate, a loss of employment and public humility since some cities post the names in the arrest in the local newspaper.

If they stick with what we can hope to be **a legal hand release,** then everyone is safe, **and the law is on their side.**

The first thing is to separate a hand release from intercourse or mouthing on genitals (blow jobs) as we know those two activities are the kind that might break up a marriage or relationship and have health concerns since some people wouldn't use protection.

So, we have to change the verbiage of the law and the people will adhere to the new law.

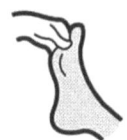

~~~~

A mention from Vermont in this Forum:

http://www.datehookup.com/thread-1352528.htm
Happy endings are actually legal in Vermont. You see, over the past 2 years, Asian massage parlors have been popping up like mushrooms in Vermont.....this is because of a loophole in Vermont's laws dealing with prostitution. The Vermont laws specifically state that sexual intercourse or oral sex in return for payment is illegal. However, the Vermont laws say nothing about happy endings in return for payment being illegal.

Thus, the Asian massage parlors have been expanding their operations in Vermont.

In order to stop people from massaging in cars, boats, trucks and public bathrooms, public outdoor areas, etc. we should set the law books straight from the beginning. If we set the verbiage in the laws books to read: **A hand release is legal when it is included in a massage situation in a massage parlor, salon, spa or fitness center.   And we need a separate category for Body Rub people with perhaps less training required and who would also be able to give a hand release.**

~~~~
This article will support the need for a legal hand release on many levels.

https://www.thestar.com/news/gta/2007/09/11/parlours_manual_release_ruled_legal.html

# Parlor's 'manual release' ruled legal

By **NICK PRON** Courts Bureau
Tues., Sept. 11, 2007

Around the Newmarket courthouse, they're calling it the "Monica Lewinsky ruling," a reference to the White House intern who performed a certain sexual act on then-president Bill Clinton.

Although that was an oral act, the case in the courthouse north of Toronto that is creating such a buzz involves "manual release," and whether or not masturbating a client at a Vaughan body rub parlor was an act of prostitution.

Justice Howard Chisvin, of the Ontario Court of Justice, didn't think so, and dismissed two bawdy house charges against Valeri Ponomarev, the manager of Studio 176, in a recent ruling that said: "The payment of money was for a full-body massage. The act of masturbation was optional, at no additional fee. I wonder, and I am left in doubt as to whether or not the community might consider the act of masturbation in all situations to be sexual."

The judge then made a reference to Clinton's liaison with the intern.

"One only needs to look to the conduct of a certain president of the United States and ... the activity that he participated in to wonder whether or not the act of masturbation is indeed, in all circumstances, a sexual act."

Will the judge's ruling open the flood gates for more "happy endings" at rub and tugs without fear of police prosecution?

Lawyer Alan Gold says it's too early to tell. But he said he believed the judgment to be unprecedented and said it will be in the next issue of his *Criminal Law Netletter*, a collection of "novel and important" cases.

In his ruling, Chisvin was critical of the undercover York Regional police officer in the case.

The court heard how the officer stripped naked, lay first on his stomach and then flipped over for the female attendant, stopping her when she put her oiled-up hands on his penis.

He went to the massage parlor again, going through the drill with another attendant.

"It strikes me that his actions were not only unnecessary but outside a protocol of investigative techniques of offences of this nature and bordered on no more than attending for self-gratification."

~~~~

Another relevant article:

Urban Dictionary: Titled Hand Release
http://nb.urbandictionary.com/define.php?term=Hand%20release
TOP DEFINITION

Hand Release

A hand release is a sexual technique usually done by a masseuse or masseur on a person by stimulating their erect penis to produce an orgasm and ejaculation. A hand release can also be done on a woman by stimulating her clitoris to produce an orgasm.

A hand release after a massage is called a "happy ending". A release before a massage is called a "happy beginning".

There are different types of hand releases. The most common is the "hand job" – stroking of the penis to produce orgasm. A "French" release is a blow job. A "Swedish" or "Russian" is a release done between a woman's large breasts.

Hand releases on males are usually done after the massage – the therapist uses a lubricating solution to stimulate the erect sexual organ. Massage oil or cream is usually used, but other sexual water based lubricants, such as Astroglide or KY Jelly can be used.

Institutions that are involved with massage education and licensing are very much against hand release during a massage session because in many places it is illegal and can be termed as a form of prostitution. However, it is very hard to arrest a masseuse or masseur for giving a hand release; and although the act of hand release is considered illegal it is rarely if never found out by the legal or licensing authorities.

Licensed massage therapists usually don't do hand releases because of legal or ethical reasons, but there are many professionals who don't see anything wrong with them and will gladly do them once they get to know you better or for an extra fee. Massage therapists have to be very careful when they offer a hand release out of fear of being caught and arrested by an undercover police officer. This is rare though.

"Do you want a hand release?" the buxom Russian massage therapist named Olga asked me.
av Melinda Goldberg 10. oktober 2004

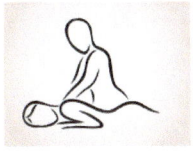

~~~~

Another relevant article:

http://samadimd.com/sexual-health/2015/12/7/health-benefits-of-hand-jobs

SEX LIFE
HEALTH BENEFITS OF HAND JOBS

December 07, 2015 Dr. David Samadi

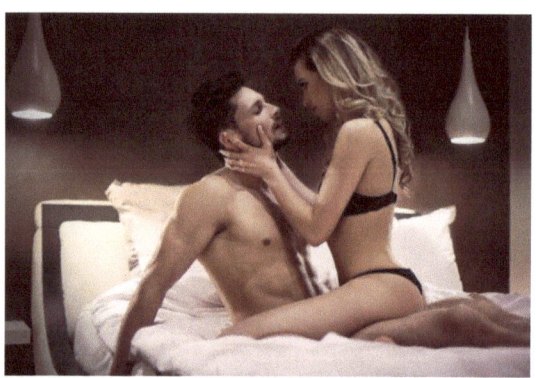

Hand jobs might get a bad rap as being weird or gross to talk about, but masturbation can help both men and women remain sexually active as they age. Like any other tissue in the body, the sex organs need exercise. Getting regular and maximum blood flow to these areas can keep the tissues and arteries healthy and functioning as they should. Masturbation can help protect the nerve fibers and blood vessels responsible for erectile function.

Masturbation can also be advantageous because it helps men, and more especially women, recognize for themselves what feels best during stimulation, including differences in speed and pressure of self-pleasure. Knowing what feels good can help you verbalize your sexual needs with your partner and have a more fulfilling sex life.

How do hand jobs benefit men?

·   Help improve immune system functioning

·   Promote prostate health

·   Build resistance to prostate specific infections

·   Some research has said masturbation lowers a man's risk for developing prostate cancer

How does masturbation benefit women?

·   Helps improve immune system functioning

·   Helps build resistance to yeast infections

·   Helps relieve pre-menstrual symptoms (PMS) like cramps

·   Increases pelvic blood flow and reduces backaches and pelvic cramping during menstruation cycles

·   Relieves headaches

·   Can help relieve chronic back pain

·   Can increase a woman's threshold for pain

What are the best health benefits of self-pleasure for both men and women?

·   It strengthens pelvic floor muscles, leading to better vaginal wall tone and harder erections

·   Form of stress relief

·

Releases endorphins (happy hormones) and can boost mood

· Can act as a sedative for better sleep

· Can increase energy levels

· Can protect you against sexually transmitted diseases, as it is a form of safe sex practice

In general, why is sex even manual pleasure, good for couples?

· Sex is exercise: Sex is an excellent form of physical exercise. It may not be as optimal as getting a proper workout in the gym, but it still helps. During sex, we burn about five calories per minute. It also increases your heart rate and uses muscles that we don't regularly use. Having sex on a regular basis can be a great addition to your regular workout routine.

· Sex lowers risk of heart attack: Having sex on the regular is good for your heart. It is an excellent way to increase heart rate, as well as help keep estrogen and testosterone levels in balance. If you have a low heart rate or your estrogen and testosterone levels are out of whack, you may be at risk for serious health conditions like heart disease or osteoporosis. Research has shown that men who had sex at least twice a week were half as likely to die of heart disease as men who had sex rarely.

· Sex lowers blood pressure: Research has found that there is a link between sex and lower blood pressure. Previous studies show that sexual intercourse lowered systolic blood pressure.

· Sex increases your libido: The more you have sex, the more you will want it, and the better it will be for you and your partner. For women, having more sex increases vaginal lubrication, blood flow, and elasticity. All of these make sex feel better and make it more desirable.

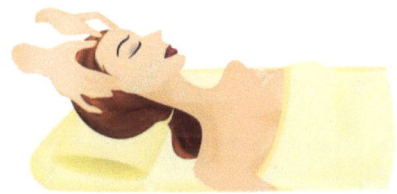

Image Essay

Please enjoy our Image Essay that with a whimsical, light hearted view you can see the many benefits that will be derived from the legalization of a hand release during a massage experience.

Fight "Procreation Pressure!" Think about Legal Hand Releases during a Massage.

The legal part needs some work. Yes, sex workers, legislators, massage business owners and the massage customers all must shout with joy that an answer has come to the oldest profession, the answer is modern limits.

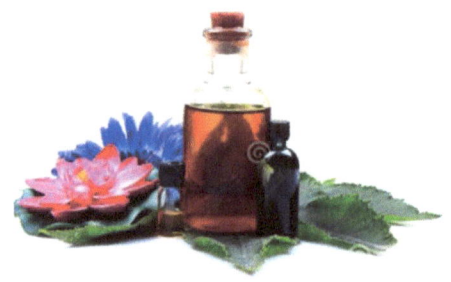

Limits will enable everyone to be happy. Just a hand release with your massage or just a massage, it's an option.

The masseuses have talent and will relax your whole body, mind, and spirit.

They've got music!

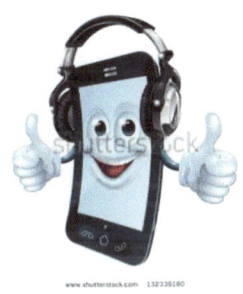

They've got massage beds, towels, oils and refreshments.

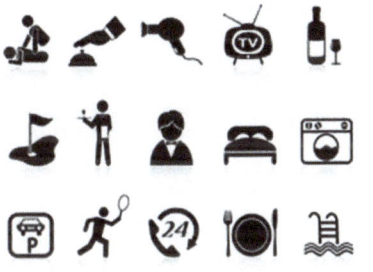

They've got rocks, the massage rocks, candles, incense, and flower petals.

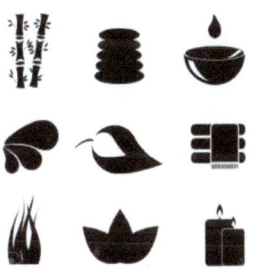

All kinds of massage parlors would participate.

Oriental Massage Parlors would be glad to gear up.

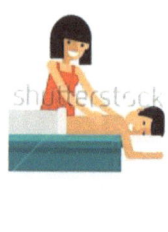

Swedish Massage Parlors would bring their kind of deep tissue relief to the situation.

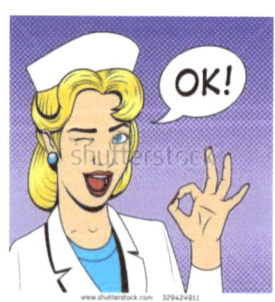

Russian Massage Parlors would tub, rub, and release.

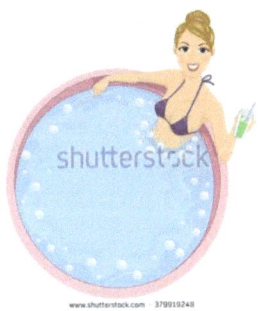

East Indian and other Massage Parlors would welcome the new business.

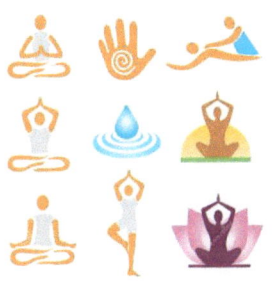

People of all skin colors, ages, status, and religion would want to get a massage.

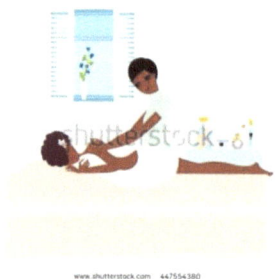

There would be no stopping the amount of new friendships and
healthy activity that a legal hand release would create.

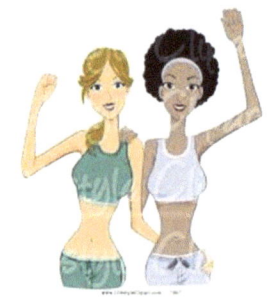

Best of all more jobs would be created for Men and...

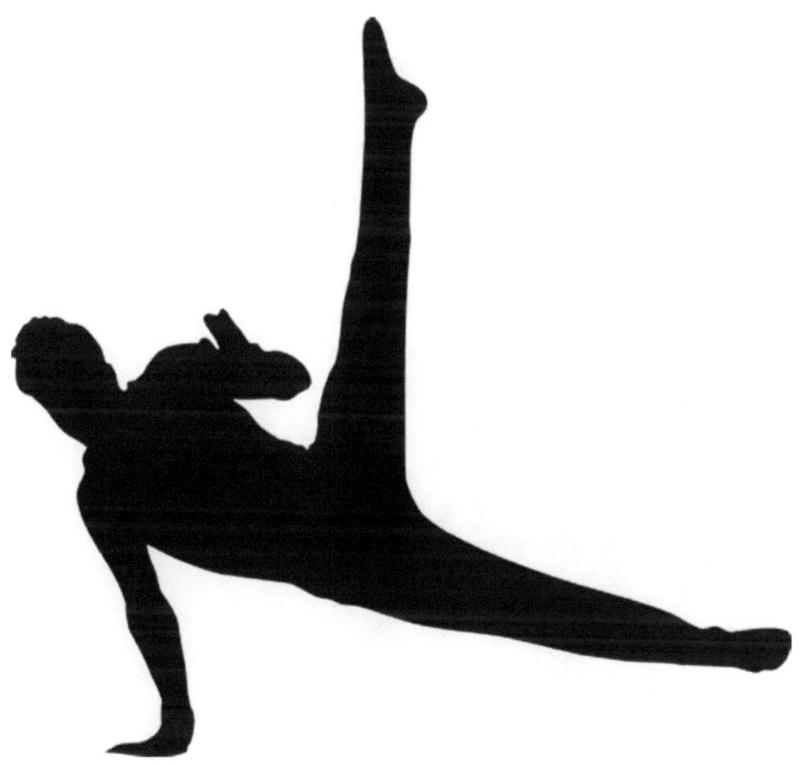

For Women!

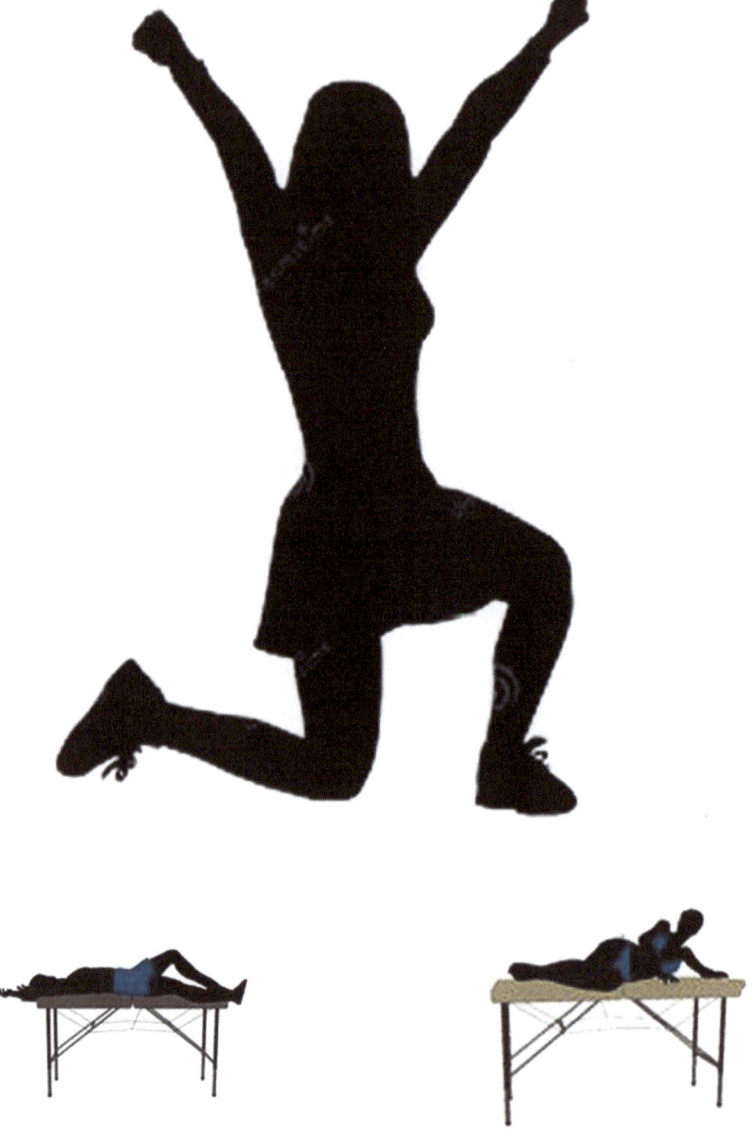

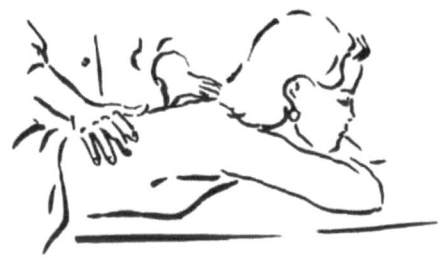

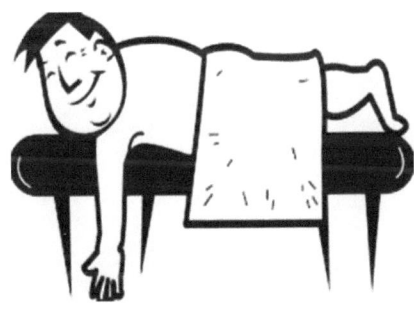

Couples get massages together and when they are apart. A hand release won't stop couples from having fun in all they do; in fact they will be happier without the "procreation pressure!"

Stop "Procreation Pressure"
Legalize a Hand Release Today!

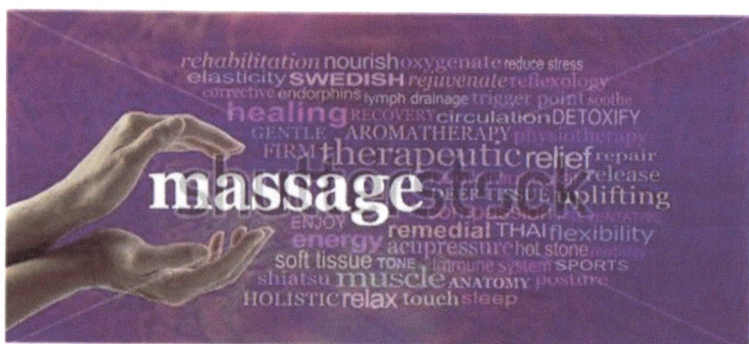

Summary

As mentioned on Page 1...

Survival, the uncanny ability that through selection a person, thing or idea stays worthy and with life in it.
The time has come: we need a legal hand release situation.
And for the time being, consider the self pleasure ending.
Another book by Phila Vocia
**Massage
with a
Self Pleasure Ending**
By Phila Vocia

Hello again. I am Phila Vocia:

This book is an addendum to my book More Massages Please - Massage with a Legal Hand Release 2016.
It is a proposal and suggestions so the eager business owner or new entrepreneur or Massage Therapist, to open this type of massage parlor, salon, spa or fitness center or add this service to their existing business and provide this service. Note that currently Massage Therapists have to have a Massage License in the USA.

I have done a lot of research.

You can assume that I have worked in the sex industry for over 20 years. I know what I am talking about.

In that time, I have not seen one piece of national legislation that makes, sex or a hand release a legal activity.

The sexy people are forced into having illegal activities to meet the biological needs of their bodies.

It's a rather inhumane environment of sexy stimulation from movies, TV, general magazines and the porn industry. The stimuli is so great that people really are walking around wondering when, where and will I have sex.

We know that major religions frown on birth control.

Many governments frown on paying for birth control.

Many life mates don't want to go against their church and do extra sex that doesn't lead to a baby. Hence many life mates seek their sex outside of their relationship and wind up in illegal activities.

What is a person supposed to do if their life mate won't have sex with them?

I suggest that sexy massage parlors with a self-pleasure ending will meet the demand, and help all the sexy people have a safe, clean environment to do self-pleasure.

Here are suggestions for the type of Massage Parlor that I know will attract business.

Please check with the local zoning board as to what permits you need for a massage parlor.

If you want to sell sex other massage items like videos and lotions check that zoning as well. You can also have vending machines. One for beverages, one for snack bars, chips and cookies etc. one for lotions, aspirin, toothpaste, mouthwash etc.

If you already have a massage parlor, you can do it if you check the zoning rules about vending machines etc.

You can do it at a new location, like near a convention center, airport, bus station or other designated business district.

Visit some popular massage parlors, get a massage. Some advertise sensual massage. Try some individuals who do sensual body rubs.

To avoid using closed circuit TV, your clients could do their self-pleasure in the restroom or on the massage table and you could leave the room for a while. Make sure you provide paper towels, wipes and the same in the restroom.

OK here is the easy part: Put it all together. Envision this or any combination: The massage parlor has colorful dim lights, soft sensual music, a few little candles and or incense burning or both. Clean wipes, and a bathroom with paper towels and soap are a must.

A massage licensed gal or guy is ready to o the massage.

A gal in perhaps could wear anything that is comfortable and complimentary to your body shape.

A gal in perhaps could wear anything that is comfortable and complimentary to your body shape and appealing.

I think if a cross dresser would want a massage, be a masseuse you would just proceed the same as with anyone else.

Next a sensual massage would take place, back to front but without touching genitals or the anus. Applying lotions can be optional. After about a 40-minute massage the customer can lay quiet and do self pleasure. Have paper towels in the massage room and in the bathroom.

Give complimentary face masks or sunglasses from the dollar stores or other inexpensive brand to the client if they wish to wear them during their self pleasure.

Example: Charge about $100.00 for a 1-hour massage plus tax. Pay your masseuses, perhaps $60.00 plus tips you keep $40.00 per massage. Cut it in half for a half hour rate. Perhaps you can have 2 or 3 massage rooms? Calculate how many massages you would like to occur in a week and how much a starter inventory of extras would cost. The sales of other items is recommended to increase profits. Then seriously consider opening this type of salon.

Any sales of optional massage elements, toys, lotions, and essential oils for example are up to you.

There is a need. We need to meet the demand.

Think about it. Do your research.

Above all, have fun.

Before you shake your head or run away,

consider these few points:

Biology, the study of how natural elements combine

Anatomy, the study of your physical form

Sociology, the study of people interacting

Anthropology, the study of learned behavior

Survival, the uncanny ability that through selection a person, thing or idea stays worthy and with life in it.

The time has come we need a legal hand release situation.

End of Massage with a Self Pleasure Ending

Thanks for purchasing our book. More Massages Please!
Massage with a Legal Hand Release
Tell a friend about us or give this book as a gift. Follow the
Author on Facebook and Twitter and see our websites, send
us a note:

Phila Vocia Author Page Link

https://www.amazon.com/stores/author/B00MX1DI4Y/

Facebook

https://www.facebook.com/PV-Author-Page-510206509431946/

Inspirational, by Phila Vocia

www.colorsass.com

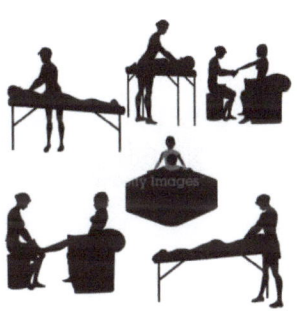

The End